D0856144

What Do You Use To Help Your Body?

Maggie Explores the World of Disabilities

✳✳✳

By Jewel Kats

Illustrated by Richa Kinra

Author's Site: www.JewelKats.com

Library of Congress Cataloging-in-Publication Data
Kats, Jewel, 1978-
What do you use to help your body? : Maggie explores the world of
disabilities / by Jewel Kats ; illustrated by Richa Kinra.
p. cm. -- (Growing with love series)
ISBN-13: 978-1-61599-083-2 (alk. paper)
ISBN-10: 1-61599-083-6 (alk. paper)
ISBN-13: 978-1-61599-082-5 (pbk. : alk. paper)
ISBN-10: 1-61599-082-8 (pbk. : alk. paper)
1. Self-help devices for people with disabilities. 2. People with disabilities I.
Kinra, Richa, ill. II. Title.
HV1569.5.K37 2011
681'.761--dc22
2011012658

Distributed by Ingram Book Group (USA), Bertrams Books (UK)

Loving Healing Press Inc.   www.LHPress.com
5145 Pontiac Trail   info@LHPress.com
Ann Arbor, MI 48105

Tollfree USA/CAN: 888-761-6268
London, UK: 44-20-331-81304

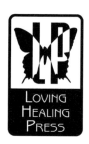

Dedication:

For my mommy, who walked me to school in the rain.
For Roopali, who is as sweet as Maggie.

Maggie hops, skips and J-U-M-P-S over bumpy pebbles sitting in her way.

"What will I learn about on today's walk, Momma?" Maggie asks.

"For today's outing, I've arranged something special," Momma says. "You'll meet people who use different things to help their bodies."

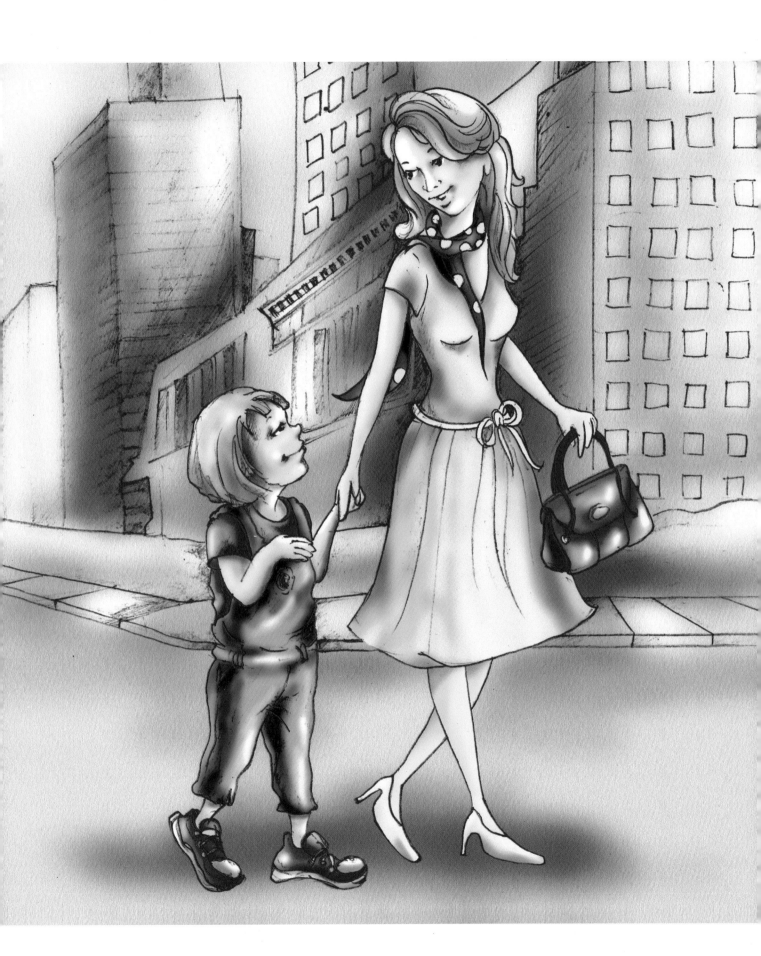

Maggie and Momma stop to chat with, Liz, who sells fresh flowers on the street.

"What do you use to help your body?" Maggie asks.

"I use a hearing aid," Liz says showing off her ear. "It helps me listen to voices and sounds coming from near and far."

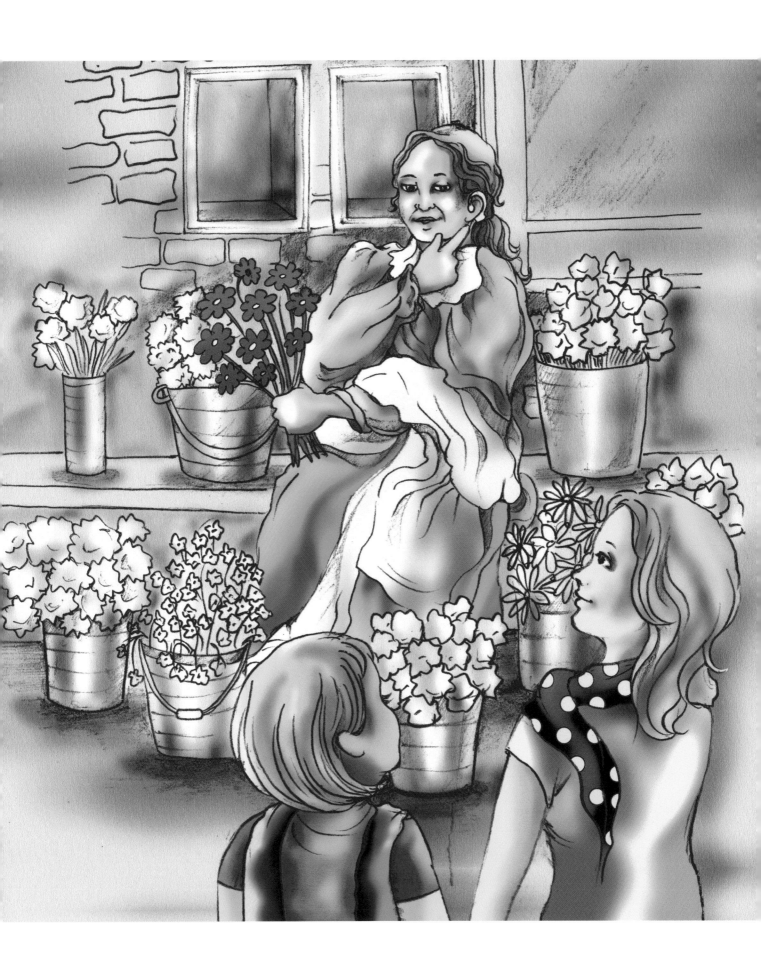

Maggie and Momma stop to chat with, David, who's getting off a Para Transit bus.

"What do you use to help your body?" Maggie asks.

"I use a wheelchair," David says. "It helps me zoom around school and home even though I can't stand or walk."

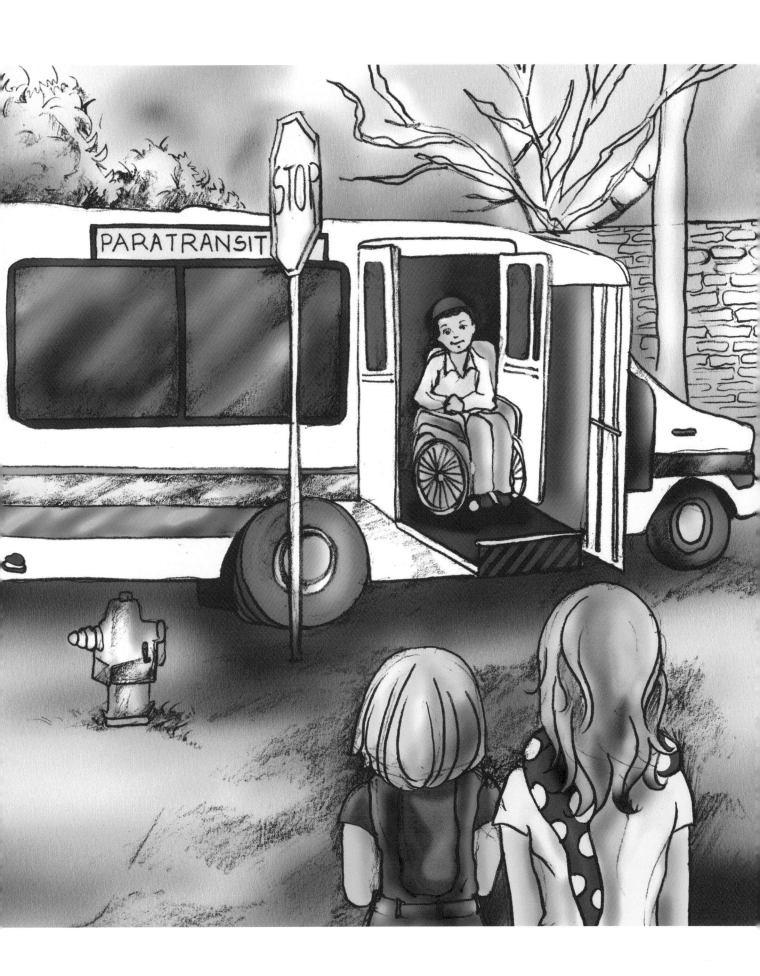

Maggie and Momma stop to chat with, Justin, who teaches a hip-hop dance class at the park.

"What do you use to help your body?" Maggie asks.

"I use an artificial leg," Justin says lifting up his pants. "It helps me stand, walk and bop."

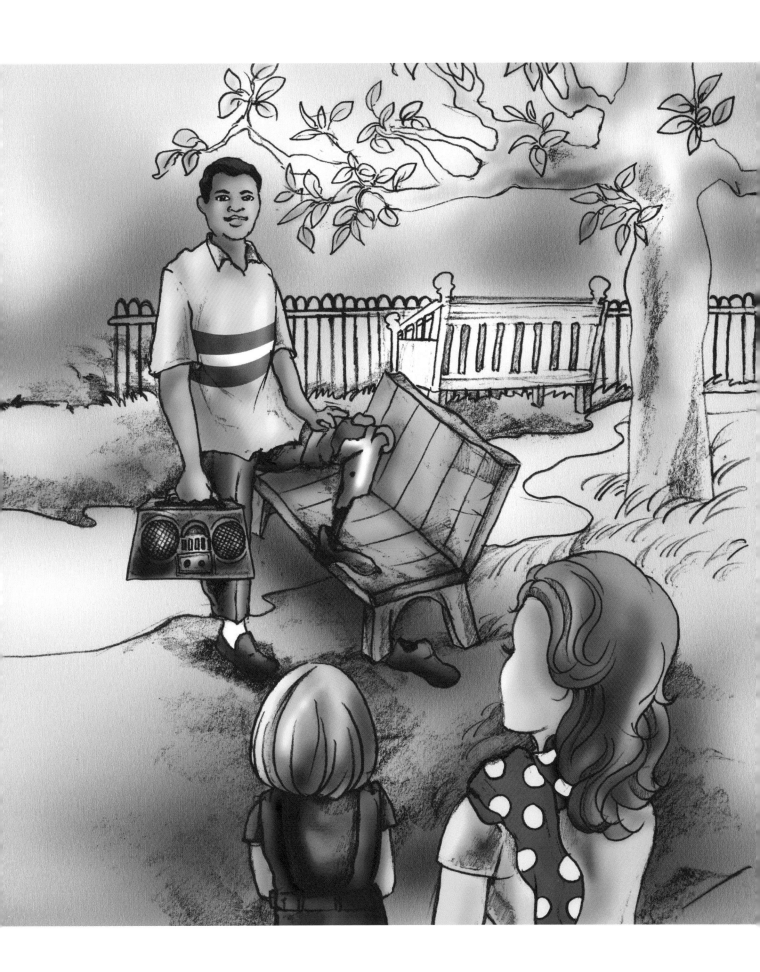

Maggie and Momma stop to chat with, Mrs. Ali, who writes poetry under trees.

"What do you use to help your body?" Maggie asks.

"I use a walker," Mrs. Ali says. "It helps me move on my feet, and I can sit down on my walker's seat when I need to relax."

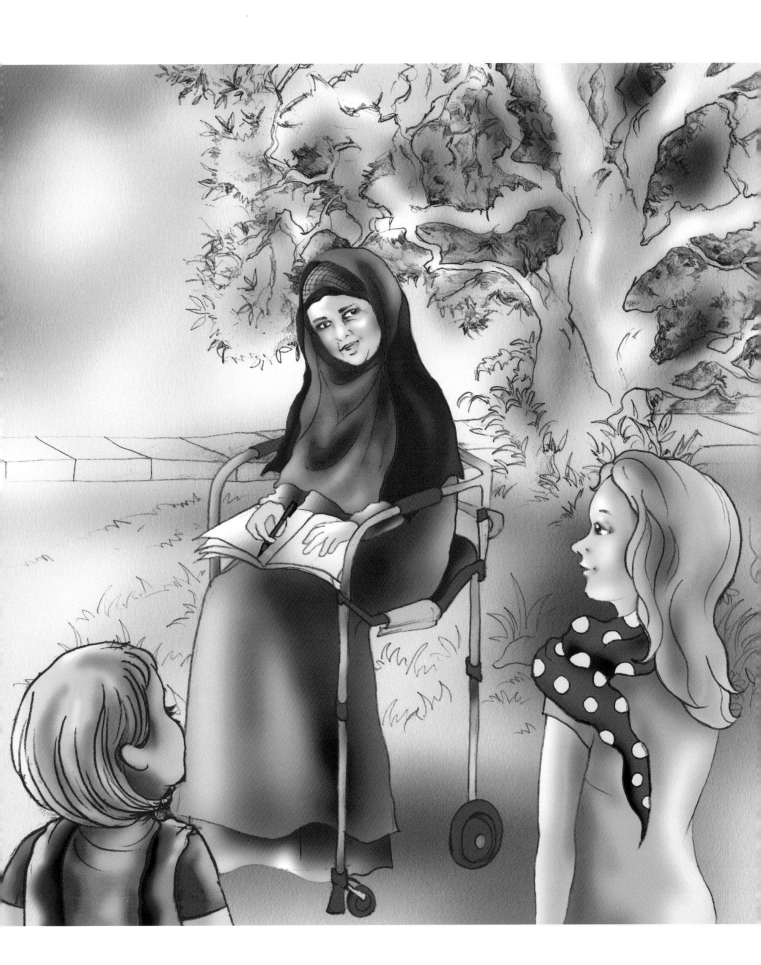

Maggie and Momma stop to chat with, Yan, who paints by the lake.

"What do you use to help your body?" Maggie asks.

"I use a communication board," Yan explains. "I can't speak clearly. So I point to the pictures and alphabet on my board to spell out what I need and think."

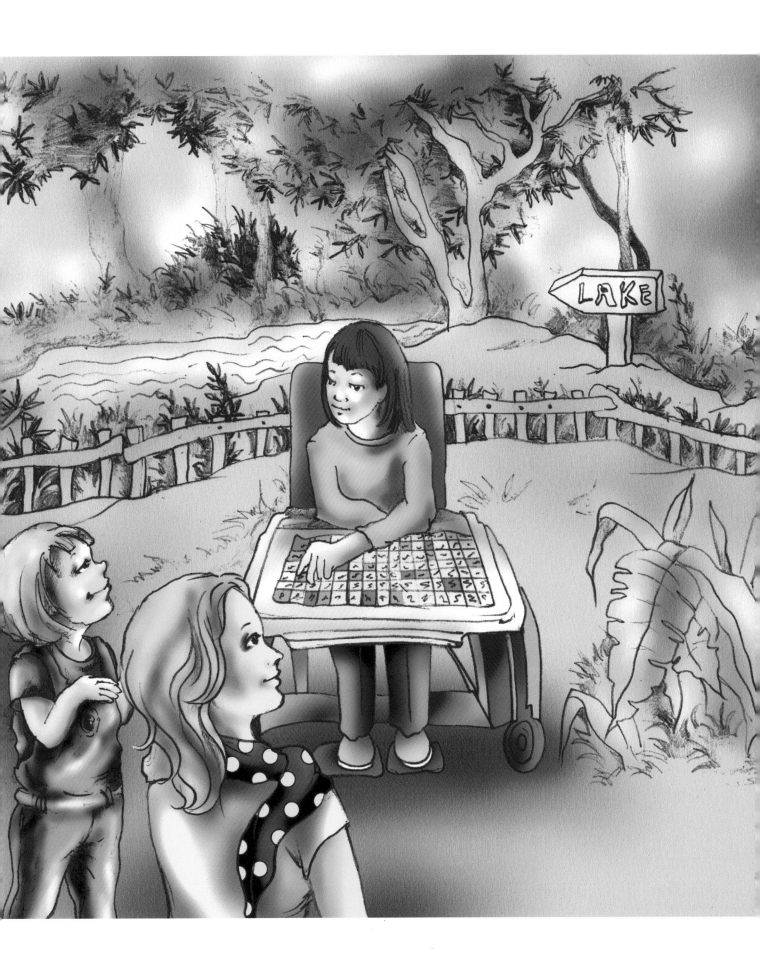

Maggie and Momma stop to chat with, Dr. Sharma, who's enjoying a tomato and cheese sandwich at a picnic table.

"What do you use to help your body?" Maggie asks.

"I use a cane," Dr. Sharma says. "It helps me stay balanced while I walk, and I use it to keep weight off my leg."

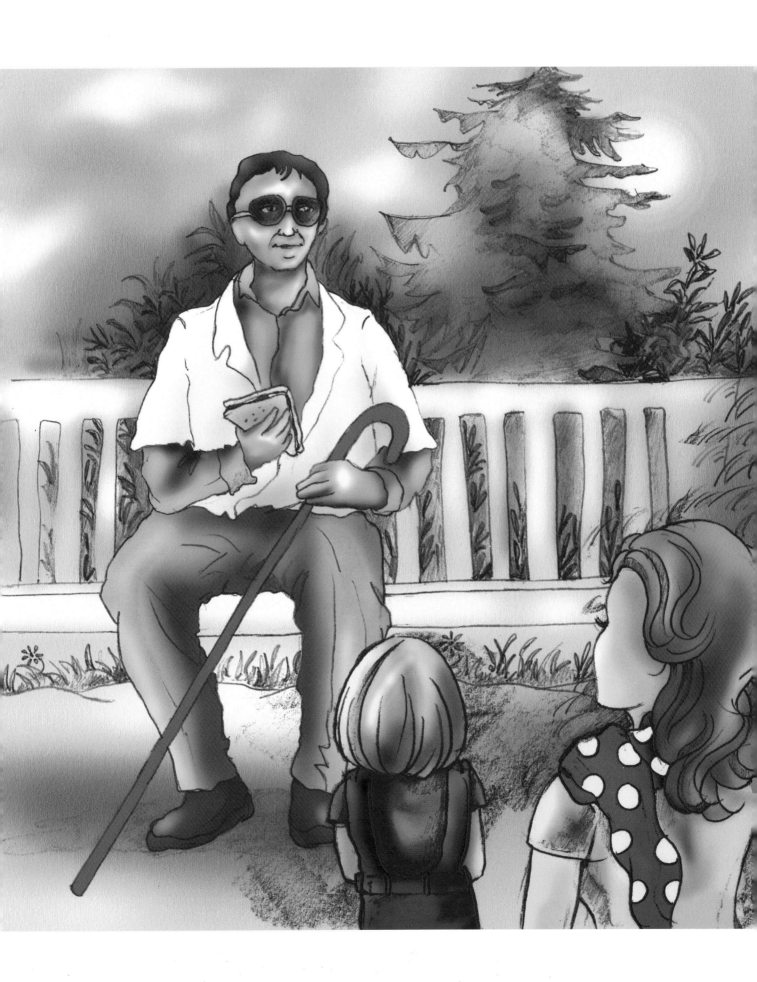

Maggie and Momma stop to chat with, Todd, who's waiting at a traffic light on his way to band practice.

"What do you use to help your body?" Maggie asks.

"I use a guide dog," Todd says. "I'm blind, and I use my trained animal to help figure out if a path is safe. Remember, you shouldn't pet guide dogs while they work. They need to pay attention."

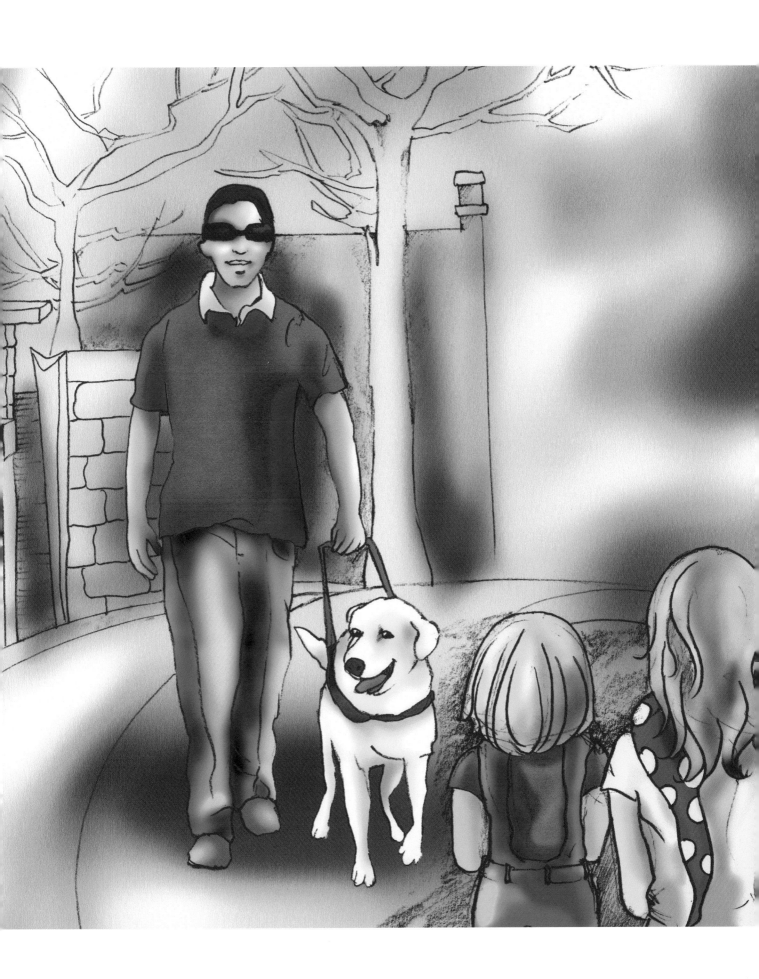

Maggie and Momma stop to chat with, Katrina, who works as a crossing guard.

"What do you use to help your body?" Maggie asks.

"I use an arm brace," Katrina says. "It helps keep the pain away, and makes it much easier to bend my elbow."

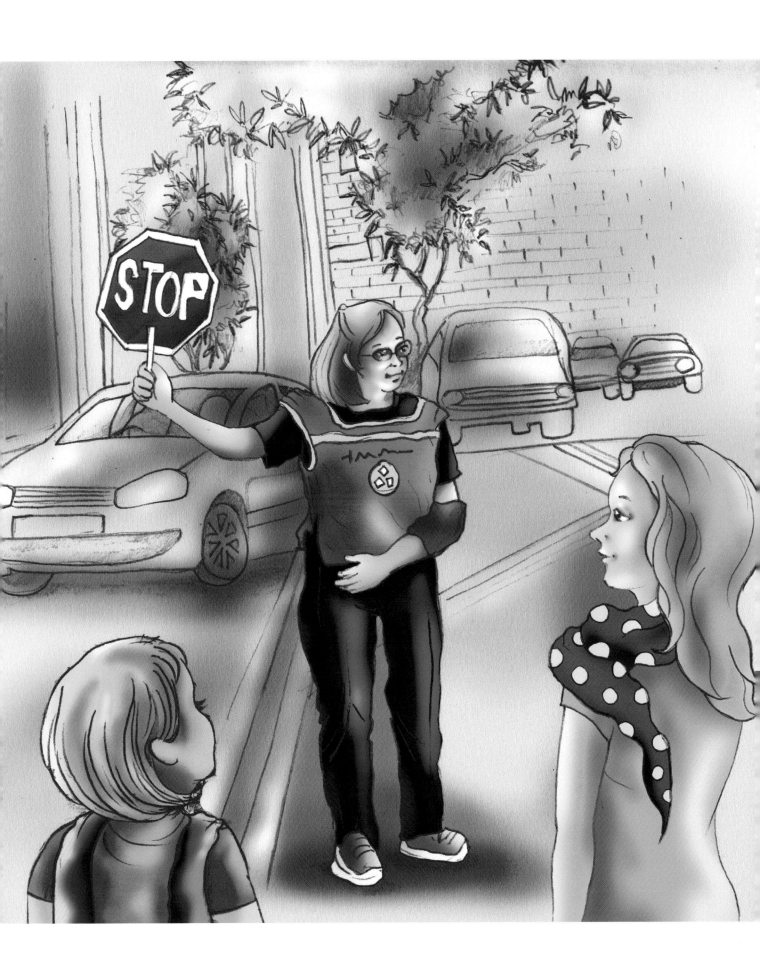

Maggie and Momma now arrive back at their home.

This time, Momma asks: "What do you use to help your body, Maggie?"

"I use an eye patch," Maggie answers. "It helps strengthen my eyesight, and lets me see beautiful things like you!"

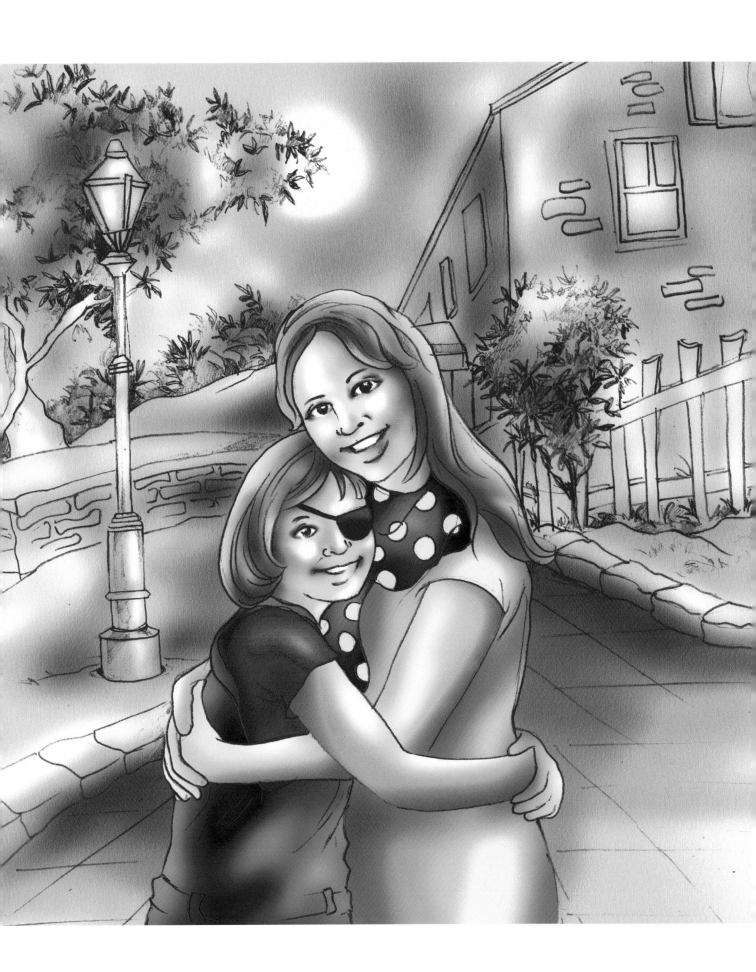

After a long elevator ride up, Maggie and Momma enter their cozy apartment.

"Do you know what the grownup word is for things that help your body?" Momma asks.

"No, I don't know," Maggie says, wiggling out of her shoes. She bounces onto her feet. "Please tell me, Momma!"

Momma smiles. "They're called 'assistive devices.'"

"Neat!" Maggie shouts. "Now, I can ask grownups about their 'assistive devices' all the time."

"I'm afraid not, Maggie," Momma says "Not all people are comfortable talking about their disabilities."

This time Maggie smiles. "That's okay. I'll be respectful like you taught me."

Momma tousles Maggie's hair. "That's my girl. I can always count on you to see things right... Eye patch or not!"

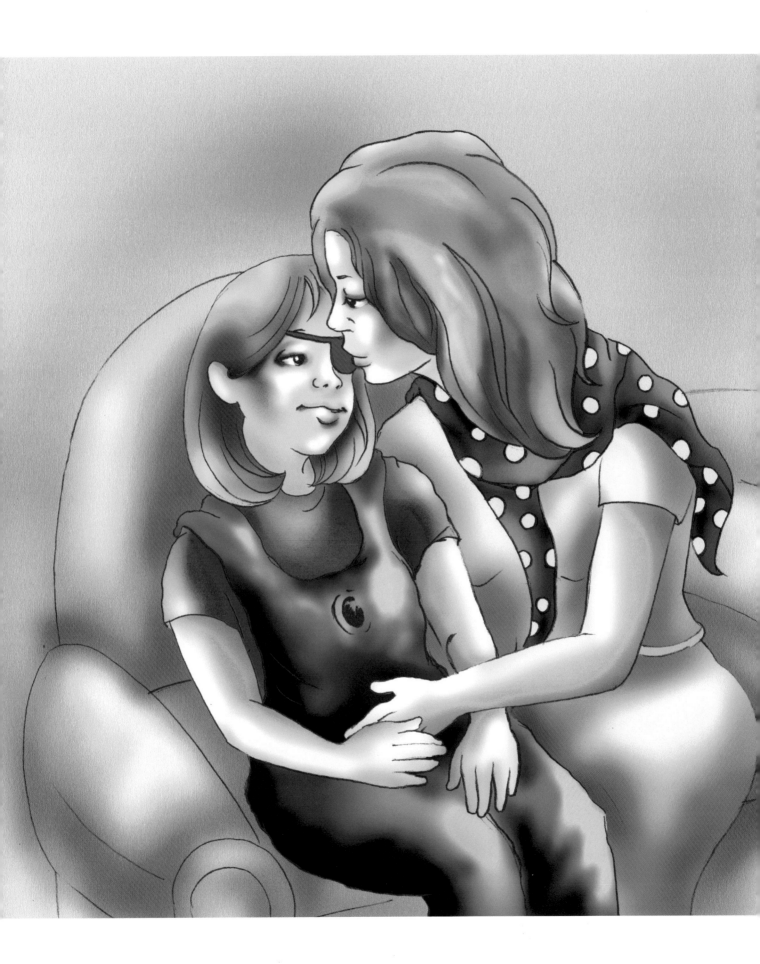

AUTHOR BIOGRAPHY

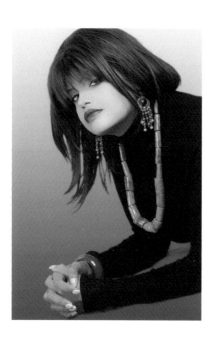

Jewel Kats (1978 –) is an award-winning writer. For six years, she penned a teen advice column for **Young People's Press**. "Confidentially Yours" appeared in dozens of newspapers via the **Scripps Howard News Service** and **TorStar Syndication Services**. Her work on this column led her to win a $5,000 writing scholarship by women's publisher, **Harlequin Enterprises Ltd.** She later earned a $15,000 scholarship from **Global Television Network**.

Jewel's first children's book is called: "Reena's Bollywood Dream: A Story About Sexual Abuse." She is excited about her forthcoming picture book: "Cinderella's Magical Wheelchair." Jewel hails from an Indo-Canadian background, and calls Toronto home.

Jewel's website: www.JewelKats.com
Contact info: JK@JewelKats.com

Richa Kinra (1984 –) is the internationally published illustrator of several children's books, adult fiction books and spiritual poems. Her books include titles such as Annabelle's Secret: A Story About Sexual Abuse, Will the Courageous: A Story About Sexual Abuse, Debra meets her best friend in Kindergarten. She is from India. She lives with her family, and says she received a lot of encouragement from her parents and friends who saw her artistic talent. Apart from children book illustrations she has also freelanced for various magazines and websites. Her hand painted works are primarily in watercolors, acrylic and oils, sometimes incorporating colored pencil, dry colors, pen & ink and/or collage.

Richa's Website:
http://www.coroflot.com/pinkdamselblack
Contact Info: richa.kinra@gmail.com

Other great titles in the Growing With Love Series

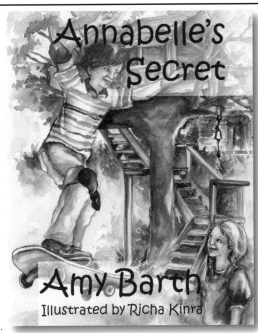

Annabelle has a secret. When she was seven years old, she was approached by a neighborhood boy and invited into a "secret club". A few years later, when Annabelle turns eleven, she finds some bad feelings have returned for her.

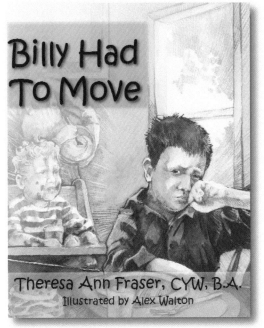

Child Protection Services have been involved with Billy and his mother for some time now. He has been happily settled with his grandmother. As the story unfolds, Billy's grandmother has unexpectedly passed away.

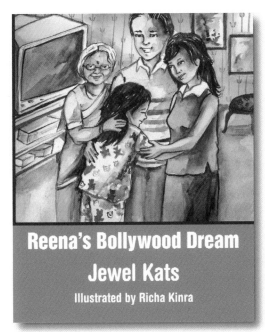

8-year-old Reena wants to be a star. Unfortunately, her family won't stand for it. However, a beacon of hope arrives in the form of Uncle Jessi. Reena is surprised by Uncle Jessi's inappropriate requests when they are alone.

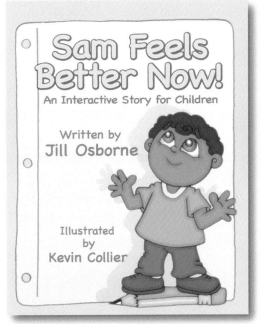

Sam saw something awful and scary! Ms. Carol, a special therapist, will show Sam how to feel better. Children can help Sam feel better too by using drawings, play, and storytelling activities.

...from Loving Healing Press
www.LHPress.com/growing-with-love

CPSIA information can be obtained at www.ICGtesting.com
Printed in the USA
BVIW12n0706180117
473509BV00013B/22